THE VITAMINS EXPLAINED SIMPLY

In the nineteenth century food contained all man's nutritional requirements, but today the vitamin content of food is dangerously diminished by processing and chemical additives. This book reveals what ailments vitamins prevent and gives estimated daily requirements of each vitamin.

THE VITAMINS
EXPLAINED SIMPLY

●

*Prepared and produced by the Editorial Committee
of Science of Life Books*

●

SCIENCE OF LIFE BOOKS
4-12 Tattersalls Lane, Melbourne, Victoria 3000

Fifth Edition, revised and reset, 1971
Second Impression 1972
Sixth Edition, revised and reset, 1975
Second Impression 1976
Third Impression February 1977
Fourth Impression October 1977
Fifth Impression 1978
Sixth Impression 1979

Registered at the G.P.O., Sydney for transmission through the post as a book.

National Library of Australia card number and ISBN 0 909911 68 1

Typeset by Specialised Offset Services Ltd., Liverpool and printed and bound in Great Britain by Richard Clay (The Chaucer Press), Ltd., Bungay, Suffolk

CONTENTS

ABBREVIATIONS USED IN THIS BOOK

mg   milligram
ug   microgram
i.u. international unit

WHAT VITAMINS ARE

During the nineteenth century, various research workers recognized, from experience gained with scurvy, rickets, and beri-beri, that there were certain unknown factors in food, capable of preventing these diseases.

Experiments were conducted to ascertain what the mysterious food factors were. In these experiments, all the then known constituents of food, namely, re-purified fat, protein, carbohydrates, mineral salts and water were fed to laboratory animals under test conditions.

Prof. J.C. Drummond, in *The Englishman's Food*, says:

'There was a good deal of interest about that time in the function in the body of the various mineral salts derived from food. Prof. Bunge of the University of Basle, Switzerland, was particularly interested in the subject and in 1881 he encouraged a young Russian assistant, N. Lunin to attempt to rear young mice on food mixtures that had been so purified that they contained very small residual traces of mineral salts. Not surprisingly, he found that they suvived a very short time.

' ... Finally he added the whole of the mineral ash of milk, thinking that by doing so he would be supplying all the necessary minerals. To his surprise the results were no better. ...

'Side by side with these cases of mice were others containing animals fed on milk itself. The animals flourished.

'Bunge asked the question, "Does milk contain, in addition to protein, fat and carbohydrates, other organic substances which are indispensable to the maintenance of life? It would be worthwhile to continue the experiment". Unfortunately, Bunge did not do so. . . . He was on the very threshold of the discovery of vitamins, for it was by almost identical experiments that 25 years later, Pekelharing, Stepp, and Hopkins independently got evidence of the existence of a new class of dietary essentials.'

There seems little doubt that the discoveries by Louis Pasteur in the realm of microbiology, made public about that time, unwittingly steered many scientists away from the real cause of scurvy, rickets and beri-beri; namely, vitamin deficiencies, so that instead of searching for vitamins they were looking for microbes.

Vitamin Research Continues
The word 'vitamin' was coined by the Polish chemist Casimir Funk in 1911. He extracted from rice polishings a crystalline substance capable of curing beri-beri and named it 'vita-amine', meaning essential to life and health and containing basic or 'amine' nitrogen. Subsequently, the final e was omitted and the word became 'vitamin'.

Up to the present, over twenty different vitamins have been isolated and more are being investigated.

Research has proved that food contains minute quantities of substances required for normal growth and the maintenance of health. These substances are now known to be vitamins, which may be defined as essential food accessories.

How Vitamins are Destroyed
In 1906, Sir Gowland Hopkins postulated the existence of what he called 'accessory factors' in foods, and between 1913 and 1920, three of the substances, namely, vitamins A, B and C were isolated.

Vitamins are thus chemical compounds which, with minor exceptions, cannot be made in the body, but come from food. Without vitamins, as we have seen, neither normal development nor health are possible.

Some vitamins are destroyed by absorbing oxygen from the air, some are destroyed by heat and water, as in cooking, and some by light. Some again, are destroyed by the presence of inorganic iron.

Dealing with this matter in more detail we find that:

Vitamin A is destroyed by exposure to oxygen.

Vitamin B_1 is destroyed by the prolonged heat of cooking.

Vitamin B_2 is destroyed by exposure to light, and is leached away in water used for cooking.

Folic acid and vitamin B_6 are destroyed by light, and the heat of cooking.

Niacinamide is lost in the cooking water.

Vitamin C is leached away after being soaked in water and is destroyed by the heat of cooking, also by fruits and vegetables becoming stale.

Vitamin E is destroyed by the presence of inorganic iron.

Water-soluble and Fat-soluble Vitamins

The vitamins are divided into two groups, namely, the water-soluble vitamins, which comprise the B complex group and vitamin C, and the fat-soluble vitamins, namely, vitamins A, D, E, F, and K.

Fat-soluble vitamins require that some fatty foods be eaten to ensure their assimilation. The use of mineral oil laxatives is dangerous because they prevent the absorption of the fat-soluble vitamins, which are therefore lost to the body.

The water-soluble vitamins are not stored in the body, but must be replaced daily.

Size Is Not Important

Because vitamins are so minute, some people may consider them insignificant or even valueless, but this viewpoint is illogical. The atom, for example, is so minute that it cannot be seen even under a powerful microscope, yet scientists have not only split the atom, but have harnessed its energy. It should be remembered too, that viruses and bacteria are extremely minute, but are able to make people sick.

Vitamins are not to be confused with drugs. Vitamins belong to the field of nutrition, and are readily assimilated. Drugs, on the other hand, *are foreign to the body* and usually have troublesome side effects, as well as destroying vitamins in the system. 'Every drug' according to Dr E.S. Bayrd of the Mayo Clinic U.S.A. 'is potentially harmful'.

VITAMIN A

It has been known for centuries that there is a substance in liver, beneficial in certain eye diseases.

In 1904, Mori treated conjunctivitis in Japan by giving cod liver oil. In 1909, laboratory rats on diets deficient in milk and butter developed conjunctivitis. By 1913 it was recognized that a fat-soluble factor was involved. This was named vitamin A by McCollum and Simmonds in 1917.

Functions of Vitamin A

Research has revealed that vitamin A has special functions relating both to the skin and that inner covering known as the epithelium. The latter lines the inside of the mouth, nose, sinuses, throat, bronchial tubes, air passages in the lungs, stomach, intestines, gall bladder, urinary bladder, kidney tubules, mastoids, inner ear, also the inner surface of the eyelids and conjunctiva.

Laboratory tests with animals have shown that when their diets are adequate in all respects except for vitamin A, they develop infections in some or other parts of the body already mentioned. Other test animals fed adequate vitamin A, remained free from these infections.

Dr Wolbach of Harvard School of Medicine, has shown that when there is a deficiency of vitamin A, the cells forming the epithelium multiply at a faster rate than normal. When these cells die, they become hard and dry. Other cells growing beneath them, push them upwards and they too die, so that presently there are layers of dry, dead cells, as occurs with dandruff.

Work of Healthy Cells

Healthy cells of the epithelium secrete a moisture that keeps growth normal, but dead cells do not. The surface of the dry cells is therefore not washed clean with mucus, but is roughened and retains bacteria in an environment favourable to their rapid growth, that is, where there is food available for them in warm, sheltered surroundings. These bacteria exude enzymes (ferments) which are toxic to the body and the enzymes break down the body's cellular structure.

Healthy cells, on the other hand, produce anti-enzymes, which destroy the enzymes released by bacteria. One of these anti-enzymes, lysozyme, is contained in the mucus secretion found in the nose and also in tears, and has a strong antiseptic action.

After vitamin A had been added to the diet of laboratory animals previously deprived of this vitamin, healthy changes in the epithelium were observed within five days. In human beings, such changes take longer, depending upon the severity of the vitamin A deficiency.

Carotene

Vitamin A is formed in the liver of humans and animals from a substance called carotene, so named because it was first obtained from carrots.

Carotene is found in yellow and yellow-reddish fruits and vegetables such as apricots, oranges, yellow peaches, melons, carrots, squash (vegetable marrow), sweet potatoes, yams, yellow corn, pumpkin, etc. It is also found in green vegetables, especially parsley, and in green pastures and aquatic plants such as seaweed, etc. There is, however, little or no carotene in white vegetables, e.g., potatoes, white turnips, cauliflower, cucumber, and white onions, nor does carotene occur in any worthwhile amount in cereal or vegetable oils, excepting soya bean oil.

As both carotene and vitamin A are destroyed by oxygen, it is inadvisable to peel carotene-containing vegetables such as carrots until just before cooking. If they are to be eaten raw, such vegetables should not be grated until actually required.

Because it is the precursor of vitamin A, carotene is known as a pro-vitamin. The relationship of carotene to vitamin A was first discovered by Moore in 1929.

When we consume fish liver oil, we are using vitamin A ready prepared for us by fish from aquatic plants containing carotene, or perhaps from the livers of fish which form the diet of other fish.

Night Blindness

Night blindness is a recognized symptom of vitamin A deficiency. There is a substance in the retina of the eye called rhodopsin (visual purple) upon which normal night vision depends. When light enters the eye some visual purple is used up and the products of such destruction bring about nerve impulses which inform the brain what the eye sees.

Replacements of visual purple, which is composed

of vitamin A and protein, are normally conveyed by
the bloodstream to the eye to make good the losses
mentioned, but if the body's intake of vitamin A is
deficient, there is a diminished supply of visual purple
and this gives rise to dim vision in a poor light, or
night blindness.

When sties form on the eye, or corneal ulcers
occur, they are indications of a vitamin A deficiency.
Severe burning and itching eyes often lack vitamin A.

Those who are over-sensitive to light or glare, may
be in need of vitamin A and many people who find it
necessary to wear sun glasses are probably deficient in
this vitamin.

Vitamin A Feeds Hair and Skin

When the diet is low in vitamin A, the hair becomes
dry and coarse and the scalp, itchy. The hair lacks
lustre and may begin to fall out; dandruff generally
forms on the scalp and the nails become brittle, peel,
or break easily.

The effect of a vitamin A shortage upon the skin is
very noticeable. The pores become clogged with dead
cells because the skin's oil glands are not functioning
properly. The pores gradually develop blackheads,
whiteheads, pimples and other skin blemishes. The
skin on the back of the forearm, also the elbows,
knees, buttocks and thighs develops small, horny
spines. Unhealthy skin, due to this cause, is susceptible to boils, carbuncles and impetigo. Cysts may
also form around such dead cells.

Practically all the body's supply of vitamin A is
stored in the liver, the small remainder being held in
the kidneys and lungs. Excess carotene is stored in
the liver and fatty tissue below the skin.

Babies store relatively less vitamin A than adults
and Dr Wolbach considers this is why they so
frequently suffer from skin rashes and infections. He

states that babies should be given fish liver oil from the first week of birth, instead of waiting until the sixth or eighth week.

Vitamin A and Internal Organs

In certain diseases, namely, those affecting the liver and kidneys, the intestines, also pneumonia, bronchitis, and other ailments of the respiratory system, the body's requirements of vitamin A are greatly increased and its reserves are rapidly exhausted.

Stone in the bladder and kidneys usually results from a lack of vitamin A, and the elimination of waste products from the kidneys does not proceed normally, for the same reason. Stone in the bladder was produced in rats by Prof. McCarrison by depriving them of appropriate amounts of butter and milk.

Vitamin A's Many Uses

Adequate vitamin A is necessary for normal growth, for the formation and preservation of healthy bone structure, the integrity of the enamel of the teeth, good appetite and the normal production of red and white blood cells. It is needed also, as we have seen, for healthy skin and mucous membrane, and for good sight. A dry mouth may indicate a lack of vitamin A. This vitamin is also considered to delay the aging process and to promote long life.

It has been found that stored vitamin A becomes more effective if up to 100 mg of vitamin E is taken daily.

In the U.S.A., according to Prof. H. Borsook, about 50% of normal children and adults are mildly deficient in vitamin A.

A baby should be given up to 1,000 international units of vitamin A daily from birth and a growing child up to 2,000 units daily. An adult requires

approximately 2,500 units a day to ensure good
health.

The dosage for elderly people can be up to double
the adult dosage, because one's requirement of
vitamin A increases with age. In sickness, the dosage
may also call for more than the daily intake, and
some eye ailments need an increased dosage until the
trouble is overcome. But, under no circumstances
should the daily dose exceed 5,000 units.

Sources of Vitamin A

The best sources of vitamin A are fish liver oil, liver,
cream, butter, egg yolk, and milk. Vegetable sources
of vitamin A are parsley, carrots, squash, sweet
potatoes, broccoli, celery, lettuce, chard, turnip
greens, spinach, kale and tomatoes. Apricots are
richer in vitamin A than any other fruit, but bananas,
oranges and yellow peaches contain Vitamin A.

It is not advisable to rely entirely upon vegetables
or fruit as sources of vitamin A, according to Prof.
Borsook, because carotene is by no means so effective
nutritionally, as vitamin A obtained from animal
sources or dairy products.

Adelle Davis points out in *Let's Eat Right to Keep
Fit* that 'Because of the stresses of modern-day living,
our nutritional requirements are extremely high,
higher for our entire population than ever before in
our history. Because our foods are overprocessed and
refined, our chances of obtaining these nutrients from
foods are extremely low, lower for our entire
population than ever before in our history.

It is regrettably true that modern foods can no
longer be regarded as reliable sources of vitamin and
minerals.'

THE B COMPLEX VITAMINS

VITAMIN B₁ (THIAMINE)

Although vitamin B_1 or thiamine was discovered as the result of a search for the cause of beri-beri (a disease not prevalent in Europe, U.S.A., or Australia) there is abundant evidence that much of the neuritis and other nerve troubles, indigestion, constipation, poor appetite, loss of weight, and chronic fatigue, so common in the nations mentioned, are due to a lack of thiamine.

Prof. Borsook states: 'a moderate deficiency of thiamine of long duration is the most important nutritional problem for the population of Europe and America.' He adds 'nutritional surveys have shown that the average child and adult in the U.S.A. and England do not receive enough thiamine. In children, this deficiency causes subnormal growth and poor appetite.' It is estimated that 95% of the people in Australia and New Zealand suffer from a partial lack of thiamine.

Function of Thiamine

The function of thiamine appears to be that of a co-enzyme, namely, the conversion of blood sugar into energy. When blood sugar is utilized in the body to produce energy, pyruvic and lactic acids are formed. Thiamine is associated with enzymes which oxidize pyruvic acid and turn lactic acid into glycogen, for subsequent conversion to blood sugar.

When thiamine is deficient in the diet, these changes are incomplete. The two acids mentioned accumulate in the tissues, particularly in the brain, nerves, heart and blood. These acids irritate the tissues and retard the body's production of energy.

Wide repercussions follow. The nerve and brain cells can 'burn' only blood sugar to obtain energy. They cannot obtain their energy from fat by itself, or from protein. In more serious thiamine shortages the nerves may be damaged. Other nerve troubles are experienced, e.g., headaches, nerviness, neuritis, irritability, etc.

The digestive processes are also slowed down because contractions of the stomach become less vigorous, hence the food is not so effectively mixed with the digestive juices. In addition, the flow of hydrochloric acid, needed to digest proteins, slackens off or may cease altogether.

To make matters worse there are diminished secretions of bile, pancreatic, and intestinal juices, all vitally necessary for a healthy digestion. Digestive enzymes, which act as ferments, are also released in smaller amounts. The net result is flatulence, gas pains, stomach trouble and poor appetite, frequently leading to loss of weight.

Constipation and Overweight
A lack of thiamine also slows down the peristaltic (wave-like) motion of the large intestine. This delays food wastes in their journey to the rectum. As a result, the faeces becomes hard and dry, giving rise to constipation, which may lead to the more serious condition called haemorrhoids.

It is known that overweight is often due to a shortage of thiamine. This is because starchy foods are only partially converted into energy owing to a paucity of enzymes, and tend to be stored as unwanted fat.

As less blood sugar is available for conversion to energy, the overweight person tires easily, soon becomes breathless, suffers from palpitation and generally has a craving for sweets — which are absorbed without being broken down by enzymes. Sweets give a temporary 'lift', but later on, result in a steep drop in the level of the blood sugar, causing fatigue and mental depression.

Thiamine and the Heart

Thiamine plays an important part in maintaining the health of the heart and its rhythm. Experiments with laboratory animals reveal that when thiamine is inadequate, the heart is the first organ to be affected. A thiamine deficiency initially slows down the heart beat and as this vitamin lack becomes more serious, the heart muscles, hampered by an accumulation of pyruvic and lactic acids, become irritated. This causes the heart to race and may result in heart failure. In all types of heart ailment it is prudent to ensure an adequate supply of thiamine.

In their book *The Avitaminoses*, Drs W.H. Eddy and G. Doldorf state: 'Thiamine deficiency impairs the function of the heart and increases its tendency to fluid collections. Dr J.S. McLester in *Nutrition and Diet in Health and Disease* confirms the above. He says 'a thiamine deficiency causes a degeneration of the heart muscles'.

The Brain and Thiamine

Persons whose intake of thiamine is inadequate, suffer from poor memory, lack of initiative, confused thinking and frequently from depression and fear. The reason is that the brain cells depend upon blood sugar for their energy and blood sugar, as we have remarked, cannot be transformed into energy without thiamine. Moreover, the accumulation of pyruvic and lactic acids which follows a poor supply of thiamine, has a toxic effect upon brain cells. Tests carried out by American medical scientists put this matter beyond doubt.

Thiamine Removed from Wheat

Thiamine is almost wholly extracted from wheat in

the milling process. Prof. J.C. Drummond in *The Englishman's Food* states: 'By 1890 the change in the character of the national diet, which attended the displacement of the centuries-old process of grinding flour between stones by roller mills, was complete. ... The gravely deficient "poverty diet" of England, which persisted throughout the thirties dated from about 1890 and was responsible in the last decade of the nineteenth century for a marked deficiency in the physique and physical efficiency of much of the community.'

Thiamine is removed from all white flour products; it is virtually absent from most packeted and processed cereals and biscuits, also from white sugar, jellies, margarine, jam, polished rice, tapioca, and soft drinks, which make up a proportion of the everyday dietary.

Prof. Drummond continues: 'Many foods contain moderate amounts of vitamin B_1, but none has a very high concentration. The richest natural source is yeast. Wheatgerm and other unprocessed cereals, as well as bran are good sources. Other sources are peas, beans, egg-yolk, liver, kidney and pork.'

Because thiamine is water-soluble, like other B complex vitamins, it is not stored in the body and must be taken daily to ensure good health. This vitamin is vulnerable to heat, air and water in cooking. Only a minimum of water should be used in cooking and it should first be brought to boiling point and the lid kept tightly on the saucepan to exclude air. Cooking soda partly destroys thiamine in vegetables and is never used by conscientious cooks.

Requirement

According to Adelle Davis in *Vitality Through Planned Nutrition* the daily requirements of thiamine advisable for health are:

Adults, 5 mg; children, 1 to 3 mg, according to age. In marked thiamine deficiencies, larger dosages are required, but dosages of the order of 50 mg and more daily, should only be taken when directed by a physician.

VITAMIN B₂ (RIBOFLAVIN)

In 1879, a research worker named Blyth obtained from whey a substance which he named 'lacto-chrome', but not until 1932 was it suspected that this natural, water-soluble, yellow-green fluorescent pigment, which occurs also in plants and animals, was a most important factor in nutrition.

In 1932, Warburg and Christian isolated from yeast a yellow enzyme. Other investigators were seeking to discover the function of this enzyme in nutrition, and in 1933 it was isolated by Kuhn and his co-workers and proved to be riboflavin (vitamin B_2).

By 1935, Karrer and Kuhn, working separately, had successfully completed the synthesis of riboflavin.

The effect of riboflavin deficiency was noted by Stannus in 1911 when he described a group of symptoms, including sore tongue and lips, sores at the corners of the mouth and in other parts of the body, now recognized as a riboflavin deficiency. Stannus considered that these lesions were caused by dietary deficiencies, but nothing was then known of riboflavin.

Laboratory rats deprived of riboflavin developed eczema and baldness, and their eyelids became gummed and affected by conjunctivitis.

Function of Riboflavin
One function of riboflavin is to aid in utilizing

carbohydrates, i.e., to turn the sugars and starches we eat, into energy. Riboflavin combined with protein and phosphoric acid, forms enzymes needed for the breaking down of blood sugar and its conversion into energy. Riboflavin is concerned with at least five different enzymes and is essential to life. Relatively large amounts of this vitamin are stored in the liver and kidneys and a certain level is maintained in the tissues.

Like other B complex vitamins, riboflavin is soluble in ater. It is lost by perspiration and urination. Although unharmed by oxygen and the heat of cooking it is leached away in the water used for cooking.

Exposure to light destroys riboflavin, thus a bottle of milk left standing in bright daylight loses most of its riboflavin content within a few hours. In strong sunlight the destruction is much more rapid.

Sources of Riboflavin

Riboflavin is contained in milk, yeast, liver, and leafy vegetables. It is also supplied in heart, beef muscle, veal, chicken, apricots and tomato. There is little riboflavin in cereals and legumes and in fish liver, while fish flesh contains virtually none. Beer contains significant amounts of riboflavin.

Deficiency Ailments

A dietary deficiency of riboflavin can arise from several causes, namely, faulty habits of eating, food faddism of the 'I don't like salads' type, over-use of alcohol, and restricted diets for such ailments as stomach ulcers, colitis, diabetes, etc. In addition, some people do not assimilate riboflavin completely, owing to a lack of hydrochloric acid in the stomach.

According to *The Vitamins in Medicine* the following ailments can result from a shortage of riboflavin: the lips burn, become red and fissured, sometimes crusted (cheilosis); the tongue becomes inflamed, fissured and burning and there may be difficulty in swallowing; there is cracking, scaliness and softening at the corners of the mouth (stomatitis). There may be seborrheic (greasy) dermatitis, pimples and flushing of the face. The nervous symptoms include numbness, burning feet, muscular weakness, dizziness, nystagmus (rolling of the eyeballs); difficulty in walking, tremor or shaking, and mental apathy.

Eye Complaints

The eye ailments arising from a lack of riboflavin include roughness of the eyelids, watering, sensitivity to light, blurred vision, dimness of sight, conjunctivitis, burning of the eyes, twilight blindness, disorders of the cornea, retrobulbar neuritis, inflamed iris, and dilation of the pupil.

Tests have disclosed that adult laboratory animals will die on a riboflavin deficient diet and growth can be slowed or stopped in young animals. Female animals deprived of riboflavin, may produce deformed offspring.

Requirement

The amount of riboflavin needed for health are 1 to 4 mg daily for children, according to age and 4 to 5 mg daily for adults. Adolescents need a full adult dosage.

VITAMIN B₃ (NIACIN)

Niacin, known variously as niacinamide, nicotinic acid, and nicotinamide, was discovered by Huber in 1867, but its significance in nutrition was not realized until 1938 when Kuhn and Vetter isolated it from heart muscle and Frost and Elvehjein discovered that it had growth-stimulating properties.

Niacin occurs in all living cells. It forms part of the body's enzyme system and promotes oxidative processes and the transport of hydrogen atoms.

For the last two centuries, the disease known as pellagra, from pelle agra, meaning rough skin, has occurred fairly constantly in districts where maize is the staple item of food.

It is now known that maize is deficient in tryptophane, an essential amino acid which is a precursor of niacin. The conversion of tryptophane to niacin is considered to occur in the tissues, not as a result of the action of intestinal micro-organisms.

Niacin is present in almost all the tissues, chiefly as a co-enzyme and more is contained in the liver than any other organ. Chronic alcoholics and those with serious liver ailments, may have difficulty in storing niacin because of this fact.

Niacin is resistant to the oxygen in the air and also to the heat of cooking, but like riboflavin, it is easily leached away in the water used for cooking.

Sources of Niacin

The foods richest in niacin are liver, meat, fish, yeast and wheatgerm. Other foods containing niacin are eggs, nuts, and wheat bran. There is practically none in white flour. Niacin deficiency can be produced by the use of sulphanilamide drugs, also by antibiotics such as penicillin.

Research into the nutritive properties of niacin followed investigations as to the cause and cure of pellagra, a disease which affects the skin, intestinal tract and nervous system.

Pellagra

A comprehensive study of pellagra was made in 1725

by the physician Don Gaspal Casal in the province of Asturias, Spain, where this disease was first recognized. Further studies were made when it later occurred in the Austrian Tyrol and Rumania, where the people lived on diets containing almost no flesh foods or cheese.

Towards the close of the nineteenth century, the connection between pellagra and an inadequate diet was obscured by the development of the new science of microbiology, because as we have stated earlier, there was a tendency to ascribe every disease of unknown cause to the action of a micro-organism. This view was shared by the eminent Italian scientist Lombroso, and valuable research time was lost.

Search for its Cause

In the U.S.A. Dr Joseph Goldberger, who in 1915 was investigating pellagra for the Public Health Department, noticed that in three public hospitals in the Southern states, the disease did not spread from patients to staffs despite the absence of any special precautions. He also observed that the hospital staffs had a more varied diet than the inmates, because staff members supplemented hospital fare with food from outside, a privilege denied to patients.

Goldberger became convinced that pellagra could not be a communicable disease, but was due to the hospitals' inadequate dietary, mostly cereals. He therefore requested that a supply of meat, tinned salmon, eggs, etc., be made to the inmates, and after this improved diet pellagra was eliminated from these institutions.

It is now recognized that economic conditions influence the food supply and provide conditions for the development of pellagra, as this ailment rarely occurs among those who enjoy a varied diet, including ample protein. Pellagra mostly affects poor people, who have to exist on a limited choice of foods, lacking protein.

Niacin Deficiency Ailments

In a mild deficiency of niacin the tongue is usually a bright red at the tip, but further back, it is coated. A furred tongue and bad breath often indicate a lack of niacin. When canker sores and small ulcers form on the cheeks or under the tongue there is every likelihood that the niacin intake is inadequate.

A mild lack of niacin causes digestive disturbances, because the secretion of hydrochloric acid in the stomach falls away and stomach trouble follows. As this acid is required to promote the assimilation of protein, iron and calcium, anaemia and nerve disorders can result.

With the digestive system disorganized, food is not properly absorbed causing flatulence, constipation or diarrhoea. Gradually the entire intestinal tract becomes inflamed, to be felt noticeably in the region of the rectum and anus. Unless this condition is rectified, it may lead to colitis.

A deficiency of niacin can also cause dizziness, insomnia, irritability, nausea, vomiting and recurring headaches. In more severe deficiencies, there is a sensation of strain and tension with deep depression, which may cause the sufferer to either cry or feel like crying.

Requirement

Nutritional authorities consider that an intake of from 20 to 30 mg daily of niacin is needed by adults to maintain health, and that children require 4 to 15 mg daily, according to age.

VITAMIN B$_6$ (PYRIDOXINE)

In 1934, Gyorgyi reported having discovered a nutritional factor (distinct from the water-soluble factors then known) a lack of which caused a particular type of dermatitis in rats, somewhat resembling pink disease in infants. This new factor was called vitamin B$_6$ and was isolated in 1939 by several different investigators. In the same year, the vitamin was synthesized by Kuhn in Germany, and by Harris and Folkers in America.

Sources of Pyridoxine
Pyridoxine is widely distributed in foodstuffs. Yeast, liver, rice, and wheat polishings, peas, beans, lentils and peanuts are rich sources of pyridoxine. Fish is a moderately good source, while milk and vegetables contain little.

Research indicates that pyridoxine comprises a group of compounds. One of the group, i.e., pyridoxal phosphate is known to be active as a coenzyme.

What Experiments Revealed
Experiments with laboratory animals have revealed that skin lesions, anaemia, cardiovascular ailments, fatty degeneration of the liver, kidney trouble and nerve lesions have resulted when the animals were kept on diets deficient in vitamin B$_6$.

Dr H.H. Schroeder of the Dept. of Internal Medicine, Washington University School of Medicine, St. Louis, U.S.A., states that too little pyridoxine in the diet of experimental monkeys produced hardening of the arteries and a deficiency of this vitamin in rats caused high blood pressure.

It was noted in some instances that the antibody formation in test animals was defective and that there was increased susceptibility to infection, e.g., pneumonia.

About half the pyridoxine content in wheat is lost during the milling process; and the pasteurizing of milk, and the cooking of food can result in substantial losses of this vitamin. Both heat and light affect pyridoxine adversely.

The function of pyridoxine appears to be that of assisting the body to assimilate protein foods and fats.

Pyridoxine and Human Ailments
According to *The Vitamins in Medicine*, vitamin B_6 has been used clinically with benefit in the more serious types of neuro-muscular ailments, i.e., muscular dystrophy, Parkinson's disease, disseminated sclerosis, etc. Davis states that nervous tics and tremors respond well to pyridoxine. This vitamin has given good results, both in the treatment of nausea and vomiting in pregnancy, and when arising from irradiation sickness.

Pyridoxine seems to play an important role in the health of muscular tissue and nerves.

Probable Requirement
The probable human requirement of this vitamin is considered to range from 2 to 3 mg daily. Even in massive dosages, pyridoxine is relatively non-toxic.

VITAMIN B_{12} (CYANOCOBALAMINE)

In 1926, Minot and Murphy showed that raw liver is curative in pernicious anaemia. Other research workers began to use liver concentrates instead of liver, and in 1948, it was announced both by Lester Smith in England and Rickes in America that they had isolated the anti-pernicious anaemia factor in pure crystalline form. It was named vitamin B_{12}, and cobalt is an essential constituent of the molecule.

Sources
Vitamin B_{12} is well supplied in liver and kidney. Meat, milk, cheese, eggs and fish are all fair sources of supply.

Vitamin B_{12} is virtually non-toxic and large dosages have been given to laboratory animals without any ill effect.

Chronic intestinal disorders can result from an impaired absorption of vitamin B_{12} and thus lead to pernicious anaemia.

The Intrinsic Factor
Castle, in 1951, showed that the stomachs of people with this form of anaemia do not produce a certain substance called the 'intrinsic factor', essential if the body is to assimilate vitamin B_{12}. Other factors which tend to nullify vitamin B_{12} are lack of hydrochloric acid in the stomach and the use of laxatives, which latter hurry half-digested food through the intestines before the process of assimilation has been completed. Still another factor which retards the body's absorption of vitamin B_{12} is a shortage of dietary calcium.

Pernicious anaemia injures the nerve cells, especially those in the spinal cord. This damage results in a jerky gait, a swaying of the body, lack of co-ordination and loss of balance.

Ailments that Respond to B_{12}
Dr H. Grabner, in an article in the *Munich Medical Weekly*, reported the following ailments as responding well to vitamin B_{12}, namely, ulcers, rheumatic diseases, and muscular dystrophy. Other ailments that

have benefited from this vitamin are bursitis, migraine, shingles and psoriasis.

According to the Journal of the American Medical Association, vitamin B_{12} is being used successfully for hepatitis (inflammation of the liver). Other reports advise of the beneficial use of vitamin B_{12} for asthma, osteoarthritis and osteoporosis (porous bones).

Vitamin B_{12}, owing to the fact that it was discovered comparatively lately (1948) is still subject to scientific research. What is known of it, however, indicates that it has a variety of uses. It is not found, even in small quantities, in plants.

Probable Requirement

The requirement of vitamin B_{12} in health is unknown, but the daily intake in food may range between 2 and 20 ug. Drs Bicknell and Prescott state that 'probably one microgram daily is sufficient for maintenance', but larger doses are needed in sickness.

Note: A microgram (ug) is one one-thousandth of a milligram (mg).

FOLIC ACID

The compounds known collectively as folic acid were discovered in 1941 by Mitchell, Snell and Williams after research work on a concentrate obtained from spinach. Subsequently, this factor was obtained from liver.

In 1944 these research workers obtained concentrated folic acid in a high degree of potency from spinach, namely, 137,000 times as active as the original product. By 1945, the successful synthesis and chemical identification of folic acid was accomplished by a group of scientists working in the

Lederle laboratories, U.S.A.

Sources of Supply

Folic Acid derived its name from the word 'foliage' and this vitamin is supplied in fresh, deep-green, leafy vegetables. Liver and kidney are also rich sources of supply. Beef, and wheatgerm contain some folic acid, but root vegetables, pork, ham, lamb, cheese, milk, corn, rice and many tinned foods are very poor sources of folic acid.

A good deal of folic acid in foodstuffs is lost during storage by exposure to light, and almost all of it by the heat of cooking.

Functions

It has been ascertained that in the absence of folic acid, the living cell cannot divide, which is its normal method of development.

Folic acid, which is closely associated with vitamin B_{12} in its functions, appears to be concerned with bringing the blood into contact with all the tissues.

Requirement

According to Drs Bicknell and Prescott, folic acid produces a feeling of well-being and increased appetite. The human requirement of this vitamin is said to range up to around 500 ug a day.

This vitamin is not effective in certain kinds of pernicious anaemia which are accompanied by nerve degeneration, particularly of the spinal cord. In such anaemias, vitamin B_{12} is generally used. Conversely, there are other forms of anaemia which remain unaffected by B_{12}, but respond to folic acid.

Deficiency Ailments

A deficiency of folic acid can give rise to any of the following ailments, namely, anaemia, diarrhoea, glossitis, (inflammation of the tongue), gastro-intestinal disorders, lack of hydrochloric acid in the stomach, and a decrease in the normal number of white blood corpuscles. Folic acid has been used with success in the treatment of anaemia associated with rheumatoid arthritis, in celiac disease (a chronic intestinal disorder of infants and children) and in disorders arising from the use of sulpha drugs.

PARA-AMINOBENZOIC ACID (PABA)

PABA was first synthesized by Fischer in 1863, but it was only admitted to the B complex family in 1940, after research work by Ansbacher.

According to Drs Bicknell and Prescott, PABA is unique in that it is a 'vitamin within a vitamin' inasmuch as it forms an integral part of the B complex vitamin, folic acid. As with other vitamins of the B complex group, the richest sources of PABA are liver, brewers' yeast, and wheatgerm. Its occurrence in foodstuffs is correlated with that of folic acid. PABA is found in meat, nuts, fresh fruits, and vegetables.

Deficiencies of PABA have occurred in humans after the administration of sulphanilamide, which obstructed the use of PABA as an enzyme and gave rise to fatigue, anaemia and skin rash.

Briefly stated, PABA appears to play an important role in normal growth, skin health, hair pigmentation and the health of the intestines.

The exact daily requirement of PABA is not yet known.

PANTOTHENIC ACID

The discovery of pantothenic acid occurred in 1901 with a substance then referred to as 'bios', but now known to be a mixture essential to the reproduction of yeast, namely, pantothenic acid.

In 1940, pantothenic acid was synthesized by groups of scientists in Germany, Switzerland and America.

This vitamin is well distributed in foodstuffs, the best sources being yeast, liver, kidney, wheatgerm, peas, soya beans and peanuts. About half the pantothenic acid in wheat is extracted in the milling process.

Functions

The work performed in the body by pantothenic acid is that of a co-enzyme concerned with the synthesis of fats from starches or proteins. Pantothenic acid also stimulates the oxidation of amino acids that are converted to pyruvic acid.

Laboratory rats deprived of pantothenic acid grew coarse, scant fur. They failed to develop and suffered ailments of the blood, lungs, and stomach. When this vitamin was lacking, the response of antibodies and phagocytes in the test animals was reduced.

Deficiency Ailments

Pantothenic acid is very effective for painful burning feet. It was used successfully during World War II on American prisoners in the Orient who developed an almost unbearably painful burning of the feet during forced labour.

There is a type of eczema due to a deficiency of this vitamin. If those with painful feet and large, beefy, furrowed tongues also suffer with eczema, it is more than likely that their dietary is deficient in pantothenic acid.

Relief from the pains of neuritis has been obtained from pantothenic acid when other B complex vitamins have proved ineffective.

Requirement

Drs Bicknell and Prescott assess the daily requirement of pantothenic acid for adults at about 10 mg. This vitamin is lost in perspiration and urination.

BIOTIN

The discovery of biotin was due to a casual observation by Bateman in 1916 that a high concentration of egg-white in experimental diets is toxic.

Subsequently, it was found that certain foods, which include liver and yeast, contain an organic substance that protects test rats against the toxic effects of 'egg white' injury.

Between 1913 and 1940 this organic substance was the subject of intensive study by Gyorgyi and co-workers. By 1936 a crystalline substance had been obtained from egg *yolk* and named biotin. From about a quarter of a ton of dried egg yolk, one milligram of active biotin was obtained.

In 1940 biotin was isolated from liver and its structure established. The synthesis of this vitamin was effected in 1943 by Harris and his colleagues and also by research scientists in the Merck laboratories, U.S.A.

Sources

Biotin is widely distributed in animals and plants and good natural sources of it are — yeast, liver, kidney, egg yolk, milk, peas, molasses and cereals. Small amounts of biotin occur in many vegetables and fruits.

Research workers have discovered that there is a basic protein in egg-white which combines with biotin and prevents it being utilized by the body. This basic protein has been named 'avidin' because of the avidity with which it combines with biotin.

After avidin and biotin have formed a complex it cannot be broken down by the body's digestive processes; only by cooking or irradiation. For this reason eggs should never be eaten raw, but always cooked.

Probable Functions

It is considered probable that biotin is required by the body to assist in the metabolism of fatty compounds, and that it also plays a part in the process of growth. This vitamin is non-toxic, even in large amounts.

Biotin deficiency can be produced in test animals, not only by feeding them a diet containing much raw egg-white, but also by administering sulphanilamides.

Deficiency Ailments

A deficiency of biotin in man causes muscular pain, poor appetite, dry skin, a disturbed nervous system, lack of energy and sleeplessness.

Laboratory animals deprived of biotin lost their fur, especially around the eyes; suffered from an itchy dermatitis, retarded growth and a spastic gait. Such animals are susceptible to heart and lung ailments. Biotin appears to be essential for reproduction and lactation in mice. Puppies fed on a diet lacking in biotin, suffered from a progressive paralysis.

Biotin is considered by some research scientists to activate lysozyme, the bacteria-digesting anti-enzyme that is found in tears, mucus and body fluids.

Probable Requirement

The daily amount of biotin required by man is not known, as one form of this vitamin, known as 'd-biotin', is synthesized in appreciable amounts within the body. *Coopers Nutrition in Health and Disease* 1968 edition, suggests that the probable requirements are from 150 to 300 mg daily.

CHOLINE

Choline has been known to science since 1849. In 1939, Best and Riddell showed that the ailment known as fatty liver could be remedied by giving choline to sufferers.

Choline appears to be concerned primarily with the use of fats and cholesterol by the body. It prevents fats from accumulating in the liver and facilitates their conversion to substances suitable for passing into circulation.

According to Bloor, fats are mobilized in the liver, but when choline is deficient, the liver is overtaxed and the body's capacity to cope with storage fats is impaired.

The prevention of a choline deficiency seems to be linked with an adequate intake of vitamin B_1 (thiamine).

Sources

Choline is present in many animal and plant tissues, good food sources being wheatgerm, liver, brains, kidney and eggs. The richest source of choline is, however, lecithin. Milk is a poor source of choline. The following vegetables contain choline, namely, soya beans, asparagus, brussels sprouts, cabbage, carrots, peas, spinach, turnips and potatoes.

Dr L.M. Morrison of the Los Angeles County

Hospital, has reported that patients suffering from coronary occlusion or coronary thrombosis have derived great benefit from being given choline, and that the amount of cholesterol in their blood decreased as a result.

The amino acid, methionine, can be converted by the body into choline; therefore a deficiency of choline can result when too little protein is eaten.

The lack of choline can give rise to dyspepsia. If long continued, this deficiency will cause permanent injury to the liver.

Requirement

According to Drs Bicknell and Prescott, very little choline is excreted by the body. The requirement of choline in the average human diet is high, namely approximately 650 mg daily.

INOSITOL

Inositol was first discovered to be a food factor in 1850, but almost a century was to pass before it was recognized as a B-complex vitamin.

Inositol appears to be associated with choline and biotin. In an experiment carried out by Dr Woolley of the Rockefeller Institute, U.S.A., in 1940, mice were given a diet that lacked only inositol. They ceased to grow and hair fell out until parts of their bodies became almost denuded of fur. After pure inositol, or the inositol contained in yeast or liver was fed to the mice, new hair grew within 18 days. Experiments with other animals gave similar results.

Sources

This vitamin is supplied in heart muscle, liver, yeast, wheatgerm, oatmeal and molasses, but it also occurs in beans, peas, grapefruit, oranges, peaches, peanuts, potatoes, spinach, strawberries, tomatoes, turnips and some other vegetables. Like choline, inositol is richly contained in lecithin.

Inositol is present in all animal and plant tissues. The highest concentration in animal tissues occurs in muscle, brain, red blood cells, heart and kidneys.

Function

As with choline, inositol aids in the metabolism of fats and seems to have some effect upon the skin and muscular tissue.

There is a high concentration of inositol in the lens of the eye and in the muscles of the heart, which seems to imply that inositol is important to clear vision and healthy heart action.

Inositol has been used with benefit by those whose hair was falling out.

Adelle Davis, American nutritional scientist, writes in *Let's Eat Right to Keep Fit* that an inositol lack is linked with coronary heart ailments, also that an inositol deficiency causes constipation, eczema and abnormalities of the eyes.

Dr W.H. Eddy in *Vitaminology* says that caffeine creates an inositol shortage in the body. Caffeine is contained in coffee and tea, and in Australia the consumption of both is very high. Caffeine is also added to some popular American soft drinks.

The probable daily requirement of inositol in man is around 1,000 mg.

VITAMIN C (ASCORBIC ACID)

The discovery of vitamin C was the result of scientific investigations made to find the cause and cure of scurvy, which plagued mankind for centuries.

In 1912 Funk postulated a scurvy-preventing vitamin, vitamin C, and efforts were made to isolate it from orange and lemon juice, which had proved most effective against scurvy.

Zilva, in 1924, obtained a 300-fold concentration and in 1928 Gyorgyi isolated vitamin C which he called hexuronic acid, from cabbage and the adrenal cortex.

The structural formula of vitamin C was established in 1933 by Haworth and Hirst who synthesized it in the same year, when it was given the more fitting name of ascorbic acid.

Vitamin C is very vulnerable to the presence of air or oxygen, but if kept dry and away from light it remains stable for a considerable time.

Sources

It appears to be present in all living tissues and is well supplied in fresh fruits and vegetables, although fruits and plants are the best sources. The richest sources are rose hips, black and red currants, strawberries, and citrus fruits. Pasteurized milk contains very little vitamin C, which is probably the reason why bottle-fed infants, who do not receive orange or tomato juice daily, are likely to develop scurvy.

Cooking destroys this vitamin, both by heat and by leaching away the vitamin in the water used for cooking. Baking soda is also detrimental to vitamin C. Hot plates and steam tables, used in restaurants to keep food hot, cause rapid loss of vitamin C.

Function

Research indicates that vitamin C is essential to form and maintain healthy connective tissue. The trillions of cells that make up the body are held together by this tissue, called collagen, and when it breaks down, not only the supporting connective tissue, but the cartilage, ligaments and walls of blood vessels weaken. This facilitates the admission of invading bacteria and viruses that cause infections. Vitamin C assists the body to deal effectively with these foreign attackers, because strong connective tissue offers a powerful obstacle. Vitamin C also strengthens their natural enemies, the phagocytes and antibodies.

The antibodies produced by the liver which help to make bacteria harmless, need vitamin C to render them vigorous and active. Antibodies also detoxify allergens which enter the bloodstream in the form of pollens, dust, dandruff, and foreign proteins in foodstuffs, vaccines and serums, giving rise to such allergies as hay fever, hives, eczema, asthma, etc.

For Bones and Teeth

Vitamin C promotes healthy bone growth and the knitting of bone fractures. When this vitamin is lacking, bones become soft, porous, or brittle and break readily after a minor fall or injury. Bone fractures heal badly when there is a deficiency of vitamin C.

Degenerative changes occur in the teeth and gums when the diet lacks this vitamin. The bone of the teeth becomes injured and the enamel is weakened. The gums become inflamed and recede from the teeth, making the latter appear unusually long. The teeth, having no firm support, loosen in their sockets and pyorrhea pockets develop at the base of the teeth, forming areas of infection.

The rate of efficiency of wound healing depends upon the amount of vitamin C and protein that is concentrated in the tissues. In diseases such as T.B. and stomach ulcers, it is imperative that strong collagen be produced, to prevent further breakdown of tissue with likely re-infection.

The Capillaries

The capillaries, hair-like blood vessels that ramify into almost every part of the body, become fragile and break down when vitamin C is lacking. When this happens, blood escapes into the tissues, bone marrow joints, etc., leading to rheumatic and other ailments.

The function of the capillaries is to carry nutrients and oxygen to the cells and to carry away waste products therefrom. When supplies of nutrients and oxygen fail to reach cells, due to broken capillaries, those cells die in a matter of seconds. Dead cells have no protection against bacteria. Instead, such cells actually foster the growth of harmful invaders of the bloodstream and enable bacteria to gain access to other parts of the body. Bacteria may thus reach the joints to cause arthritis; the kidneys to result in kidney ailments, or the heart to give rise to rheumatic heart disease.

People who bruise easily, or are subject to nose bleeding are almost certain to be suffering from fragile capillaries, which require vitamin C to nourish and strengthen them.

For the Thyroid Gland and Veins

Vitamin C is needed to maintain the thyroid gland in health and to help the body to assimilate iron, needed to ward off anaemia. According to Prof. E.V. McCollum, 'There is evidence that iron utilization is defective when the body's reserves of ascorbic acid are depleted'.

This vitamin is needed too, to strengthen the walls of blood vessels; when it is deficient the veins sag, become dilated and tortuous, which marks the onset of varicose veins.

Research workers have shown that vitamin C is particularly abundant in the adrenals, the pituitary and other glandular tissue and it seems essential for the efficient working of the endocrine system of glands and the production of hormones.

The Eyes

There is a high concentration of vitamin C in the fluid within the eyeball, also in the lens of the eye, the iris, the retina, and the cornea. Experimental cataracts have been produced in aged guinea pigs by restricting their intake of this vitamin. Josephson states that the administration of up to 300 mg of vitamin C daily to patients with cataract 'caused marked improvement'. Treatment of corneal ulcers with vitamin C is reported to have resulted in a dramatic improvement, according to Drs Bicknell and Prescott.

They also state that vitamin C has been reported to have a specific diuretic effect in cardiovascular disease. When used in doses of from 300 to 700 mg daily, it produces a diuresis (free excretion of urine) in all patients.

Vitamin C Losses

Vitamin C is lost to the body by inhaling D.D.T. as contained in insecticides and pest sprays, also by smoking, inhaling the fumes of petrol, molten lead and lead paints, cleansing solvents and smog. Several drugs cause vitamin C to be lost rapidly by excretion, namely, aspirin, the barbiturates, salicylates, sulphanilamide, insulin, thyroid extract, atrophin, antihistamine drugs, adrenaline, etc. Those who lack hydrochloric acid in the stomach cannot properly absorb vitamin C.

As this vitamin is not stored in the body, it must be taken daily. It is exreted by perspiration, urination and excessive water drinking.

The use of vitamin C has proved effective in preventing or curing chemical poisoning. It corrects the toxic action of lead, bromide, arsenic, petrol and other chemicals.

Requirement

The approximate *minimum* daily requirements of vitamin C are — babies 50 mg, children and adults 100 to 150 mg.

In sickness, these doses should be increased considerably because during infections and diseases, vitamin C disappears from the blood and urine, and the quicker this vitamin is given, the sooner can recovery be expected.

Therefore, massive doses of vitamin C, i.e., in excess of 750 mg daily should be taken (with calcium tablets to counteract the acidity of this vitamin).

Vitamin C can be used with benefit for colds, hay fever, influenza, catarrh, asthma, bronchitis, rheumatic and other fevers, infections of the eyes, ears, sinuses and tonsils and for the ailments of children, as well as for arthritis, stomach ulcers, gout, etc. It is also effective for wounds and burns and, as we have already stated for bruising and nose-bleeding.

VITAMIN D

As stated previously, cod liver oil was in use a century ago as a remedy for rickets, a disease of children and marked by faulty bone formation. In adults, this condition is called osteomalacia.

In 1918, Mellanby produced rickets in dogs by giving them an unbalanced diet and he remedied the disease with cod liver oil. At the time, it was thought that vitamin A was the curative factor in rickets. Research by McCollum in 1922 demonstrated that vitamin A given in foods other than cod liver oil, failed to cure rickets. McCollum then destroyed the vitamin A in cod liver oil by bubbling hot air through it and found that oil so treated still cured rickets, although it had no value for eye infections which normally respond to vitamin A.

In 1919, research proved that the action of ultra-violet rays in sunshine, or the light from a mercury-vapour quartz lamp were also curative in rickets.

Vitamin D was synthesized in crystalline form in 1935, and since then about twenty different forms of this vitamin have been investigated but only two are in practical use, namely vitamins D_2 and D_3.

Sources

Some vitamin D_3 more commonly known just as vitamin D is contained in summer butter and eggs, but fish liver oil is the only reliable source. Vitamin D_3 is poorly represented in other foods. The second kind of vitamin D, namely vitamin D_2 is produced by the action of the sun's ultra-violet rays or the mercury vapour quartz lamp upon the skin of humans, the hair or fur of animals and the feathers of birds.

The oil glands of the skin, under the influence of sunlight or the lamp mentioned secrete a wax-like pro-vitamin called irradiated 7-dehydrocholesterol, which is thought to be converted into vitamin D, absorbed by the skin and then by the bloodstream.

When dogs and cats lick their coats, it is considered that they thereby absorb vitamin D, as do birds when they preen their feathers.

Test rats which have developed rickets from lack of vitamin D in their diet, are cured if they are allowed to lick their coats, when exposed to sunlight.

Animals which hibernate, such as the hedgehog, do not do so when given vitamin D. Under natural conditions with the approach of winter and waning sunlight, the animal's supply of vitamin D declines.

This causes it to 'burn' less blood sugar and become torpid. Its metabolism slows down and its food consumption is very low, whereas hedgehogs given vitamin D, developed too much energy to permit hibernation.

Steenbock showed in 1924 that vitamin D_2 can be added to foods such as milk and margarine by exposing them to ultra-violet rays. They thus become irradiated. Other forms of irradiated foods are available. Vitamin D_2 is also known as calciferol.

Clouds, fog, haze, and smog prevent the sun's ultra-violet rays from reaching the earth and surveys made in cities where bad weather conditions often prevail, reveal more cases of rickets than cities which have clearer skies and more hours of sunlight annually.

Vitamin D and the Teeth

Mrs May Mellanby, wife of the scientist who produced experimental rickets in dogs, carried out extensive research to establish the relationship between vitamin D and the teeth. She found that even mild forms of rickets interfere with the normal development of infants' teeth, also the structure and shape of the jawbone, causing narrow dental arches, crooked, over-lapping, and protruding teeth, defective bite, faulty alignment of teeth, etc.

According to Davis, vitamin D helps to prevent tooth decay and plays an important part in preventing pyorrhea.

Functions

Vitamin D is considered to control an enzyme called phosphatase, which appears essential to bone formation. The function of this enzyme is to act upon fats and sugars that are combined with phosphorus and to release the phosphorus for bone-building purposes.

This detached phosphorus then forms a union with calcium brought along by the bloodstream and both minerals share in building and hardening the bone structure, which in young children is a pliable, gristly substance called collagen.

The foregoing complicated processes fail to occur when vitamin D is lacking in the diet. Instead, the enzyme, phosphatase, leaves the bone foundation and enters the bloodstream. Phosphorus is then not released from fats and sugars and is unavailable to combine with calcium, hence these minerals are not deposited in the young bones and growth may cease. Half the phosphorus in the body is normally found in the bones.

Should inadequate vitamin D be supplied, some phosphatase is present, but bone growth is slowed down and the formation of teeth is delayed and disorganized.

Importance of Vitamin D

In some respects, vitamin D is the most important of all the vitamins, for deformity of the bony framework in childhood, due to a shortage of this vitamin can cause irreparable injury which continues throughout life, because once the bones harden the 'die is cast' for good or ill.

Children deprived of calcium and phosphorus in their diet also become stunted and develop bony malformations. Following World War I and the period of malnutrition which ensued, many children in Germany and Austria showed symptoms such as curvature of the spine, bow legs, knock knees, etc. Even children in their late teens were affected.

One of the functions of vitamin D is to release energy within the body. Phosphorus carries blood sugar through the intestinal wall, as well as to the liver, which stores it as glycogen. Blood sugar is 'burned' to supply energy and when vitamin D is lacking, sugar cannot combine with phosphorus, hence energy flags.

Vitamin D and Energy

Research has shown that children who lack vitamin D burn less blood sugar and display less energy than normal children. The combination of sugar and phosphorus in the muscles is reduced and the first mentioned children lose blood sugar in the urine, and their blood contains more than normal amounts of sugar. There is thus an incomplete storage of blood sugar as glycogen, and an incomplete absorption of it in providing energy.

Davis raises the question whether some of those who crave sweets are not actually lacking vitamin D, because when the body cannot use sugar, it expresses this deficiency in a craving for sweets. It is possible too that some people who lack vitamin D during winter months, owing to inadequate exposure to sunshine or infrequent sunny days, may become short of energy for this reason.

Vitamin D is important to maintain healthy eyes. Experiments with puppies showed that when fed on a diet deficient in vitamin D, changes occur in the eyes, comparable with changes noticed in the eyes of adults and children. These alterations give rise to short-sightedness or myopia, an inability to bend light rays sufficiently.

Effect of Sun's Rays

During the winter months, owing to the sun's lower altitude, fewer ultra-violet rays reach the earth. Experiments with rats kept on diets to induce rickets, showed that only five minutes of mid-summer sun is required to keep them free from rickets, whereas almost three hours of mid-winter sun are needed.

McCollum states 'Even in clear weather, and in the country, sunlight contains no appreciable ultra-violet light, except when the sun is above thirty degrees from the horizon.'

Ordinary window glass and dark, heavy clothing exclude ultra-violet rays. Dark complexioned people do not absorb as much vitamin D as those with lighter coloured skins, and people with heavy suntan cannot absorb vitamin D. Negro children are susceptible to rickets on account of their colour.

The too frequent scrubbing of horses with soap and water can produce rickets. This is due to the removal from their skin of the provitamin irradiated 7-dehydrocholesterol. Soap has a more severe effect upon 7-dehydrocholesterol than water alone.

Bathing and Vitamin D

If people take a bath before going for a swim on a sunny day, the oils that form 7-dehydrocholesterol are washed off and no vitamin D is formed. If they do not bathe before swimming, but take a shower after their swim, the oils are washed off before vitamin D can be absorbed.

Infants suffering from rickets make no progress if they are thoroughly washed when exposed to the sun's rays. It is better to wash such children with olive oil than with soap and water.

The use of paraffin oil as a laxative prevents the absorption of vitamin D as it does with other fat-soluble vitamins, namely, A, E, F, and K. Moreover, it damages the liver, according to Drs Bicknell and Prescott. These authorities also state that fluoride (used in some public water supplies in Australia to prevent dental decay in children) retards the action of vitamin D in warding off rickets.

The best source of vitamin D, other than sunlight is, as we have stated, fish liver oil. This can be

obtained in capsule form (together with vitamin A)
by those who dislike taking fish liver oil as such.

Like other fat-soluble vitamins, vitamins D and A
are best assimilated after a meal containing some
fatty food, such as butter, cheese, milk, etc.

Vitamin B_1 has a protective action against a
possible overdose of vitamin D. McCollum says: 'The
consensus of medical opinion is that feeding vitamin
D in amounts well above the minimum levels necessary for prevention or cure of rickets, has no
deleterious effect, and that the rules should be to give
it in ample quantity to cover any possible unrecog-
nized requirements.'

Requirement

Davis, in *Let's Eat Right to Keep Fit*, states: 'Fear of
toxicity has caused the National Research Council
(U.S.A.) to recommend only 400 international units
of vitamin D daily for persons of all ages,' but studies
by Dr Johnson, of the Henry Ford Hospital, Detroit,
U.S.A., 'indicate that the adult can profit by taking at
least 4,000 units of this vitamin daily.'

However, an adequate daily dosage would be
around 500 to 1,000 units.

VITAMIN E (ALPHA TOCOPHEROL)

Vitamin E was first isolated from wheatgerm oil by
Evans and others in 1936. Its existence was fore-
shadowed as a dietary factor by Mattill and Conklin
in 1920, and in 1922 Evans and Bishop proved that it
is essential for normal reproduction.

In 1931, Goettsche and Pappenheimer demonstrated that laboratory guinea pigs and rabbits developed muscular dystrophy when deprived of vitamin E
and in 1938 Bicknell started to treat children affected

by this ailment with vitamin E. Other workers followed his example, with some success.

Vitamin E occurs as alpha, beta, gamma, delta, and three other tocopherols, but only alpha tocopherol has marked biologically active properties, the other tocopherols being virtually inert. Drs Evan and Wilfred Shute, of the Shute Foundation for Medical Research, London, Ontario, Canada, and who have conducted considerable research into vitamin E, state: 'We equate vitamin E to alpha tocopherol.' For this reason, our remarks about vitamin E in what follows, refer to alpha tocopherol specifically.

Vitamin E is rapidly and completely destroyed by rancid fats and inorganic iron preparations. One of its functions is to protect vitamin A, also the B complex vitamins and biotin against destruction by rancid fats. People with over-active thyroid glands need more than normal daily requirements of vitamin E. There is evidence that it is intimately concerned with the central nervous system.

Sources

The richest natural source of vitamin E is wheatgerm, but it is also found in the germ of other cereals and in cereal and vegetable oils. There is a small amount of vitamin E in lettuce, tomatoes, carrots, egg yolk, fish roe and nuts. Vitamin E is fat-soluble and is not harmed by cooking.

The only dependable sources of vitamin E are in foods in little general use, namely, wheatgerm, freshly ground wholemeal flour and unprocessed cereals, also cereal and vegetable oils.

Foods that Lack Vitamin E

Unfortunately, when edible vegetable oils are hydro-generated, as is the current practice, most of their vitamin E content is lost. There is almost no vitamin

E retained in the popular processed cereals. Fruit contains practically no vitamin E and this vitamin is absent from yeast, lard, cod liver oil, polished rice, refined cornmeal and white flour. Butter and cream contain almost no vitamin E. Dried and pasteurized milk may contain no vitamin E according to Bicknell and Prescott, so that artificially fed babies will receive inadequate supplies of the vitamin. These two authorities also state: 'The mothers of boys with muscular dystrophy, especially when the condition has apparently been present from birth, often give a history suggesting that during pregnancy and lactation, they themselves were deficient in vitamin E.'

Research with rats has shown that cancer tissue will not grow if placed in blood serum that is enriched with vitamin E, though in serum lacking vitamin E, it will grow readily.

During the steel-roller milling of flour, the vitamin E content is removed, which doubtless explains the tremendous increase in degenerative diseases since this method of milling was adopted, about a century ago.

Functions

According to Mattill, more vitamin E occurs in the body than any other vitamin. Vitamin E appears essential for muscular health (and the heart is a muscle); it helps to utilize fat; it is concentrated in the pituitary, adrenals, and sex glands; it prevents vitamin A, linoleic acid and possibly other nutrients from destruction by oxygen within the body, and it performs several other important functions. Mattill says of vitamin E: 'Perhaps no other of the vitamins mysteriously affects so many and so varied bodily processes.'

Vitamin E Deficient in Modern Diet

Davis points out that before wheat was milled by the steel roller process, the intake of vitamin E was estimated at from 100 to 150 mg per head daily. Today, our foods supply only a tenth of this amount, or less.

Bicknell and Prescott say that there is only from 4 to 8 mg of vitamin E in English food, and about 14 mg in the U.S.A. dietary. It is likely that Australian food is just as poor in vitamin E as American food.

Requirement

According to Horwitt, the minimum daily requirement of vitamin E is 30 mg. He has shown that anything less tends to result in haemolysis, (destruction of red blood cells and loss of haemoglobin). Other research workers, namely, Engel, Harris, and Quaife, announced some years ago that the minimum daily human requirement of vitamin E is 30 mg. Vitamin E is virtually non-toxic and can be stored very efficiently by the body.

At the 1949 World Congress on Vitamin E, it was stated that a woman's requirement of vitamin E increased ten-fold during the menopause, and that an aging person may need fifty times the ordinary inadequate daily intake of approximately 10 mg.

Used for Heart Disease

The use of vitamin E for heart disease began in 1947 when Dr Evan Shute, of London, Ontario, Canada, treated his mother, then 71 years old, who was suffering from angina pectoris and a dropsical condition of the legs and arms. After five days of using vitamin E, the anginal pains vanished and the dropsical swellings, too.

Dr Evan Shute and his brother, Dr Wilfred Shute, then began to use vitamin E for other heart sufferers and within three years had treated 4,000 patients. Eighty per cent of them obtained amazing benefit, most of them losing all the usual heart symptoms.

Many thousands of medical men all over the world are now prescribing vitamin E in the treatment of heart disease and high blood pressure, also for thrombosis, liver and kidney ailments, chronic leg ulcers, varicose veins, menopausal ills, serious burns, Buerger's disease, Reynaud's disease, and even early gangrene.

There is probably no vitamin that has lifted the shadow of despair from so many sufferers, as vitamin E.

Properties of Vitamin E

The following properties of vitamin E have been discovered:

1. It is a vasodilator, i.e., it dilates the capillaries and enables blood to flow freely into damaged, anaemic muscle tissue, thereby strengthening both the tissue and the nerves supplying it.

2. It decreases the oxygen requirements of muscle tissue by approximately 50%. This is equivalent to an enhanced blood supply and diminishes pain and breathlessness.

3. It is an antithrombin, namely, it dissolves blood clots and prevents their formation, but does not interfere with the normal clotting of blood.

4. It prevents the formation of excessive scar tissue, and in some instances even melts unwanted scar tissue.

5. It promotes urine excretion, hence is useful to heart patients with dropsical conditions.

6. It preserves the integrity of the walls of the capillaries, of vital importance to the damaged heart.

7. It increases collateral circulation, i.e., it promotes 'detour' blood channels around veins and

arteries that are blocked.

8. It lends power and efficiency to muscle tissue, and has a most beneficial action upon tired, flagging heart muscle.

An autopsy study of 300 otherwise healthy American soldiers who died violent deaths in the Korean war, showed that 77% already had coronary heart disease. Their average age was 22 years, which indicates that heart ailments are now attacking an earlier age group than ever before.

VITAMIN F
(UNSATURATED FATTY ACIDS)

The essential unsaturated fatty acids, sometimes referred to as vitamin F, were first described by Burr and Burr in 1929, when they observed 'fat deficiency' disease in laboratory rats that had been deprived of certain fatty acids.

The disease manifested in a failure to put on weight. There was also a dryness and scurfiness which spread from the paws over the rest of their bodies. Cold weather accentuated this scurfiness — the kind that chaps hands. The rats also developed kidney stones and there were difficulties in reproduction. It was observed, too, that some relationship existed between the lack of unsaturated fatty acids and two of the B complex vitamins, namely, pyridoxine and pantothenic acid.

Sources
The three unsaturated fatty acids are known as linoleic acid, linolenic acid, and arachidonic acid. These acids quickly become rancid when exposed to the air. They are found chiefly in cereal and vegetable fats and oils, namely, wheatgerm oil, safflower seed oil, cotton seed oil, rye-germ oil, maize-germ oil,

sunflower seed oil, soya bean oil, peanut oil, linseed oil, palm oil, olive oil, etc., but are poorly represented in such animal fats as butter, margarine, beef and mutton fat, lard, fish oil, or milk.

The unsaturated fatty acids evidently play an important part in the maintenance of bodily health, for they are carefully husbanded within the body.

Deficiency Ailments

A number of human disorders seem to be associated with a deficiency of these fatty acids, namely, infantile eczema, adult eczema, dandruff, boils, acne, varicose ulcers, diarrhoeal conditions and under-weight.

According to the Lee Foundation for Nutritional Research, U.S.A., unsaturated fatty acids reduce the incidence and duration of the common cold. They are also indicated when there is a dry skin, dry, brittle hair and nails, falling hair and kidney disease.

Functions

It is also stated that the fatty acids function in the body by co-operating with vitamin D in making calcium available to the tissues; by aiding in the assimilation of phosphorus, and by nourishing the skin. The fatty acids seem to be related to the normal functioning of the adrenal glands, the reproductive process, and the thyroid gland.

Cholesterol

Yet another task of the unsaturated fatty acids is to lower the cholesterol levels in the bloodstream. It is known that excessive cholesterol (derived from animal fats), tends to form deposits on the inner walls of blood vessels, thus restricting the lumen, (opening) for blood to pass through. After a time, these deposits become silted over with minerals in the bloodstream and the blood vessels harden and lose their resilience. This condition gives rise to hardening of the arteries and high blood pressure. Should a hardened particle of cholesterol break away, it may plug an important artery, causing coronary occlusion or coronary thrombosis.

Lecithin

The unsaturated fatty acids contain a substance called lecithin, also found in egg yolk, liver and brains, which appears to be a homogenizing agent, i.e., it is able to break up fats and cholesterol into tiny droplets. In short, lecithin emulsifies cholesterol, and thereby prevents it from silting up blood vessels, or forming a thrombus.

Modern Foods Lack Lecithin

You may ask why are not the unsaturated fatty acids readily available in the ordinary diet? The answer is that modern foods are processed. Many edible vegetable fats are hydrogenated to change them from oily substances to hard fats that can be cut with a knife. This facilitates handling, packing and selling, but also destroys the essential fatty acids. Vegetable shortenings, processed cheeses, some peanut butters, cooking fats and margarines receive this hydrogenation treatment.

The human body can convert sugars to fats, but it cannot manufacture unsaturated fatty acids and must therefore obtain them from the foods we eat. These fatty acids contain what might be termed chemical 'hooks' which allow other substances to be linked to them. Thus, if oxygen becomes 'hooked', the fatty acids turn rancid. Cake mixes, pastry mixes, potato chips, popcorn, and salted nuts, held too long in storage, are often rancid when purchased.

We have already seen what happens when hydrogen

is 'hooked', namely, the fatty acids harden and also lose their lecithin content. The purpose of the 'hooks' is to permit essential fatty acids to combine with other nutrients, hence they are called 'unsaturated'.

Infantile Eczema

It is suspected that many cases of infantile eczema which occur soon after birth, are due to mothers avoiding vegetable and cereal oil fats, thus depriving their systems of lecithin needed to protect the baby against eczema. Adults with eczema, according to Davis, have been found to have abnormally small amounts of essential fatty acids in their blood.

Davis states that even psoriasis, one of the most stubborn eczema-like skin ailments, responds to lecithin. This authority also points out that overweight people, whose ankles, legs and thighs are swollen with oedema, can lose unnecessary pounds after taking lecithin. It is claimed that in many instances the overweight condition is solely due to the body being waterlogged.

The Need for Fat

Bloor considers that as many obese people refuse to eat fats, the body changes sugars to fats more rapidly than normally in an effort to produce the missing nutrients. Fat people put on weight as a result and because they are usually excessively hungry they tend to overeat. It is known that fats are far more sustaining than sugary or starchy foods. Hence, by going short of fats there follows an over-indulgence in sugars and starches, both notorious weight producers for the obese.

Fat is needed to ensure the efficient production of bile, also of the fat-splitting enzyme, lipase. When fat enters the intestine, the gall bladder empties itself through a duct that leads to the intestine. Should there be inadequate fat, too little bile is formed and the faulty emptying of the gall bladder may induce the production of gallstones. Moreover, the fat-soluble vitamins, A, D, E, F and K cannot be assimilated in the absence of fat and bile, and are lost to the body.

Fat is essential to health and a small amount of stored fat is needed for several purposes. Fat under the skin protects nerves and muscles and maintains warmth in cold weather. Fat around the kidneys supports them. A fat reserve is beneficial as a source of energy during sickness. It is only when fat is too abundant that it is objectionable. It is not so much the fat you eat, but the *kind of fat* that is important.

Value of Lecithin

Lecithin, contained in safflower seed oil, soya bean oil, sunflower seed oil, etc., besides helping to keep the skin and nails in health is a rich source of two B complex vitamins, choline and inositol. It also contains vitamins E and K, and zinc. Lecithin supplies an anti-oxidant that prevents rancidity, thereby preserving from destruction the fat-soluble vitamins already referred to, together with some of the B complex vitamins in our food and in the intestinal tract.

Because it helps to form the fatty myelin sheath around the nerves which both insulates and nourishes them, lecithin is used in the treatment of nerve troubles, nervous exhaustion, and brain fag.

Lecithin is also important to the health of the intestinal flora; it aids in keeping the body free from diarrhoea and other bowel ailments.

Some people find that any kind of oil taken from a spoon is nauseating, but lecithin is available in capsule form and in lecithin granules, to make good deficiencies.

VITAMIN K

In 1931, a research scientist named McFarlane observed that fish-meal cured a haemorrhagic disease in chickens that had been fed upon diets deficient in fats. It was noticed, however, that when the fish-meal was extracted with fat solvents, no cure resulted.

It had been suspected earlier that a vitamin deficiency caused haemorrhage, and in 1934, Dam, of Copenhagen, suggested that haemorrhagic disease resulted from the lack of a fat-soluble vitamin which he named 'K' after the word 'koagulation'.

Many attempts were made to isolate the vitamin in pure form, and this was finally achieved in 1939 by Karrer, Dam, and co-workers, who obtained it in a yellow oil. Two natural forms, namely, K_1 and K_2 were identified.

Sources
Vitamin K is well distributed in green plants: alfalfa (lucerne) and spinach are rich sources of supply, but vitamin K is also fairly well supplied in cauliflower, cabbage, carrot tops, kale, soya beans, seaweed and pine needles. It is present in smaller amounts in cereals, tomatoes, honey, orange peel and bran. Most of the vitamin K occurs in the green parts of the plant. Some vitamin K occurs in egg yolk, but most animal sources are only comparable with the poorest vegetable sources. However, there is very little vitamin K in potatoes, lemon juice, most fruits, or in cod liver oil.

Without vitamin K, blood will not coagulate, but the vitamin will not arrest haemorrhage, either in normal persons, or those suffering from haemophilia (a sex-linked hereditary bleeding disease occurring in males).

Function

The sole function of vitamin K is thought to be that of a co-enzyme in the liver, to help in forming prothrombin, a water soluble protein in blood plasma. Vitamin K is stored in the liver but only in small amounts.

The coagulation of the blood is the result of a most complicated series of reactions involving prothrombin, thromboplastin, calcium, thrombin, fibrinogen, and fibrin. The actual clotting process is due to a fibrous protein called fibrin, which does not occur in the living blood, but exists in an inactive form called fibrinogen. Prothrombin in the living blood is converted to an enzyme called thrombin in shed blood. Thrombin, in the presence of calcium and the blood platelets, converts the inactive protein, fibrinogen, into fibrin. The blood clot contains corpuscles which become entangled in a web of fibrin, thus sealing off the wound and preventing further blood loss.

The precursor of thrombin, namely, prothrombin, is formed in the liver. In serious liver illness or injury, the prothrombin level in the blood falls and can endanger blood clotting.

Requirement

Human requirements of vitamin K are as yet unknown, but dietary deficiencies of this vitamin have been reported. Some vitamin K is produced by bacteria in the large intestine, but the amount is quite inadequate and must be supplemented by a dietary source of supply. The use of unsaturated fatty acids enables intestinal bacteria to synthesize vitamin K.

The new born infant during the first few days of its life, requires a supply of vitamin K from external sources, because the prothrombin level falls after birth and only returns to normal at the beginning of the second week, due to bacterial action.

Newly born babies are, therefore, subject to haemorrhage (which may occur from accidental minor injuries to blood vessels) while there is a lack of vitamin K. Brain haemorrhage can cause spastic paralysis in which the muscular movements are unco-ordinated and jerky, and the infant is handicapped for life.

For this reason, most modern hospitals give vitamin K to the mother shortly before the baby is born. The vitamin passes from the mother's to the infant's bloodstream.

Experiments with animals have shown that a rise in temperature increases the requirements of vitamin K.

A deficiency of this vitamin can be produced by the use of supha drugs, the salicylates, aspirin, and arsenical preparations.

Patients with liver ailments who require surgery, are usually given vitamin K as routine practice.

Causes of Deficiency

An inadequate absorption of vitamin K can result from a lack of bile, pancreatic insufficiency, severe or chronic diarrhoea, ulcerative colitis, intestinal obstruction, etc.

If gallstones obstruct the bile duct, the flow of bile is shut off. Sometimes the bile duct itself becomes infected, swells and closes. In the absence of bile, natural vitamin K cannot be absorbed by the intestine. This causes a lack of prothrombin and the blood may fail to clot. Synthetic vitamin K, being water soluble, does not need bile salts for its absorption.

Vitamin K is unaffected either by the air or heat, therefore leafy vegetables can be used raw in salads or cooked, as a source of this vitamin.

VITAMIN P (BIOFLAVONOIDS)

The term, bioflavonoids, refers to flavonoids possessing biological activity. The bioflavonoids are a group of carbon-hydrogen-oxygen compounds which have the property of correcting fragile capillaries and protecting their integrity. When bioflavonoids are lacking in the diet, the walls of blood vessels become porous and the red corpuscles can pass through them into the tissues, giving rise to several ailments.

The capillaries are so fine and so numerous that if the capillaries of one man were stretched out in a single line, they would reach two and a half times around the earth! We have mentioned elsewhere that the capillaries form an important part of the body's transport system and convey food, oxygen and hormones to every cell in the body, as well as removing the waste products of metabolism and disease. When the capillaries are strong and healthy, infections are quickly thrown off.

There is a growing recognition that because the capillaries are harmed in every diseased condition, there is no diseased state that cannot be helped tremendously by strengthening the capillaries.

The history of vitamin P began in 1926 when Gyorgyi and co-workers found that a substance extracted from paprika (red pepper) and also from lemon juice, was superior to vitamin C in preventing capillary bleeding.

Gyorgyi named this active substance 'citrin' and research revealed that it contained the bioflavonoids hesperidin, and the glycoside of eriodictyol. Later, other bioflavonoids were found, namely, quercitrin, quercetin, naringin, esculin, and hesperidin methyl chalcone. In 1944, another bioflavonoid, called rutin, was discovered by Griffith. Of those mentioned, hesperidin and rutin appear to possess the greatest biological activity. Rutin is obtained from a herb called buckwheat and also from eucalyptus. Vitamin P may, therefore, be regarded as a complex, similar to vitamin B complex.

Sources

The richest source of vitamin P is fruits, particularly lemons and oranges. It is in the inedible pulp and peel of these fruits, rather than the edible fruit, that vitamin P is contained. Vitamin P is also found in rose hips, blackcurrants, grapes and buckwheat.

Gyorgyi named vitamin P 'in honour of paprika and permeability', on which latter it was found to have a profound influence.

Vitamin P is readily leached out if foods containing it are cooked in water and the water is poured away. If, however, lemon peel is added to lemonade and allowed to soak, vitamin P is extracted.

Requirement

The exact human requirement of this vitamin is not known, but is approximately 50 to 100 mg daily.

Tests have shown that vitamin P enhances the biological effect of vitamin C by stabilizing the latter and protecting it against the destructive action of oxygen.

It has been shown, too, that when guinea pigs, in which scurvy has been produced, were given vitamin C, capillary fragility is improved, but still remains at a sub-normal level. When vitamin P is added to their diet, capillary integrity reaches normal level.

Vitamin P has a detoxicating action upon benzene and phenol and when used with vitamin C protects against the toxic effects of arsenical poisons. Unlike Vitamin C, vitamin P appears to play no part in the healing of wounds.

Uses of Vitamin P

It is accepted by science that vitamin P is an essential nutritional factor and that it produces a rise in capillary resistance, which cannot be obtained from vitamin C alone. Vitamin P has been used with some degree of success in diseases marked by decreased capillary resistance, namely, hypertension, rheumatic fever, diabetes, purpura, allergies, bacterial infections and toxicity arising from the use of drugs.

There is some evidence, too, that vitamin P has benefited those with rheumatism, rheumatoid arthritis, glaucoma and retinal haemorrhage, according to Bicknell and Prescott. These claims are confirmed by Martin in *Modern Nutrition in Health and Disease*.

Bioflavonoids and vitamin C have been used successfully for the common cold. A group of student nurses at Creighton University School of Medicine, U.S.A., were given tablets containing both vitamins P and C, and the results were checked against another group of nurses who received no vitamins.

The first group had 55% fewer colds and their colds lasted only half the time of those of the second group.

B complex vitamins should also be taken, to ensure normal elimination of body wastes.

Concentrates of vitamin P now available, are many times stronger than those derived from fruits.

ON TAKING VITAMINS

Davis says that the action of the B complex vitamins is synergistic, i.e., they co-operate with each other and that better results are obtained by taking them together than by taking large doses of a single B complex vitamin.

Quigley shares this view. He says: 'Physicians who have prescribed extra large doses of thiamine, have noticed muscular weakness and nervousness afterwards.' It is reasonable to expect that an overdosage of thiamine or any other single B complex vitamin would throw the other B complex vitamins out of balance, and probably nullify their activity.

Quigley continues: 'The effects of all vitamins overlap and interlace to such a degree that no disease can be cured by administering one vitamin, and no disease *is caused* by any single vitamin deficiency.'

In this doctor's experience, better results are obtained with vitamins A and D if B complex is also taken. Still better results can be anticipated by including vitamin C, and preferably, vitamin E.

We have always advised heart sufferers to take vitamin B complex with vitamin E, and vitamin C also, where indicated.

Multi-vitamin preparations are available for those who need a daily minimum maintenance dosage. Those who require a therapeutic dosage to remedy an illness, should realize that a sick person needs all the principal vitamins, but in daily dosages *larger* than a minimum maintenance dosage. Quigley states: 'Where a vitamin deficiency has existed over a long period of time, the dose that is given to correct the trouble must be several times larger than the maintenance dose.' For such people, separate vitamin capsules and tablets are available and should be taken together, in the recommended dosages.

According to Baker and Winckler, two English nutritional scientists writing in the *Medical Press*, there has been a tendency for tables of minimum vitamin requirements to be given official sanction and then to be repeatedly quoted as though they were final and absolute.